Yoga Straight & Simple

Aidan John Walsh

Sergio-Grant Kirkwood

© 2014

Content by Aidan John Walsh

Photography by Sergio-Grant Kirkwood

www.aidanwalsh.co.za

Contents

The Golden Rules of Yoga

- If it feels wrong, it is wrong, and if it feels right, it is right!
- If anything hurts, ease up a little or back out of the pose slowly!
- Avoid pain or discomfort altogether, particularly in the joints!
- Try to differentiate between good pain and bad pain! (muscular versus joint)
- Keep breathing (through the nose as far as possible). Everything else is a bonus!
- Use the breath as a guide. Strained breathing equates to strained posture. Poses should be comfortable and stable!
- Rest at any time, it's your practice so honour your own body!

Brief History of Yoga

You may not be aware but Yoga is a practice that is thousands of years old, too old to be able to say with any degree of accuracy and scholars do disagree.

Another little known fact is that there are at least three hundred differentiated Yoga methods or traditions currently practiced and recognized worldwide.

The two most prolific schools of Yoga are the Ashtanga and Iyengar schools. What sets them apart is the focus of each method.

Ashtanga is a flowing sequence of postures with less emphasis on alignment and more on cardiovascular endurance. (Vinyasa Yoga is less structured but conforms to the same principles).

Iyengar is more alignment focused with very little cardiovascular work, and more emphasis on flexibility as a healing modality. (Hatha yoga conforms more to this school as classes tend to be slower and gentler.)

Yoga developed as a holistic method of training, moving one towards spiritual awakening, and consists of eight different limbs or aspects.

What we know of as Yoga, the physical exercise including breathing exercises, are only two of these eight limbs. They are the third and fourth, called Asana (postures) and Pranayama (breath-work).

The first two limbs are about personal and interpersonal observances and ethics. The remaining four involve varying degrees of meditation practice.

We consider the other six limbs to be relatively optional as most people already have an existing spiritual practice or belief system. Some principles are still expressed in the methods of practice for both Asana and Pranayama.

What purely physical Yoga then does is help our bodies to remain strong and flexible, facilitating healing and other natural functions in the body, with the added benefit of stress reduction.

We strive for a healthy mind in a healthy body.

Breathe into It

The most crucial part of any Yoga practice is the use of the breath. As long as you're breathing, you're doing Yoga. If you hold your breath or it becomes strained, it's no longer Yoga.

This doesn't mean that Yoga should be easy. There should definitely be a sustained effort but with added emphasis and deliberate concentration on this literally, vital aspect.

Inhalation creates internal pressure on all the body organs and systems, while exhalation releases tension. Inhalation breaks up blockages and cleans organs while exhalation flushes out and softens the entire body.

The longer and fuller the breath is on both inhalation and exhalation the better. During Asana (postures) practice we aim to keep inhalation and exhalation even, breathing in for a number of seconds and breathing out for the same count.

There are Pranayama (breathing) techniques that alter the quality, length and depth of the breath and these are usually reserved for before or after Asana practice.

Ujjayi, or Victorious Breath, is the diamond standard across Yoga. It requires a soft contraction of the muscles inside the throat to create a restriction to the air flow, resulting in a sighing sound on both the in and the out breath.

The sound can be made as loud or as soft as preferred but must ideally be continuous throughout the practice.

You can imagine the sigh you might make when fogging up a mirror or glass to clean it. It is the same action in the throat but the mouth remains closed.

Breathing during Asana practice is always in through the nose and out through the nose. Inhalation through the nose warms, moistens and filters the air entering the lungs while exhalation clears the nostrils of filtered particles.

The breath is also co-ordinated to movement within Asana practice. On inhalation the spine is extended and exhalation takes you into a pose.

Inhalation typically takes place during any movement that takes you upwards, expands or extends the limbs outwards.

Exhalation typically takes place during any movement that takes you downwards, contracts or draws the limbs inwards.

The breath takes priority over the Asana in Yoga, and should fill the lungs from the top, through the middle, to the very bottom. Exhalation empties the lungs from the bottom, through the middle, to the very top.

When in doubt stop, breath, and continue on.

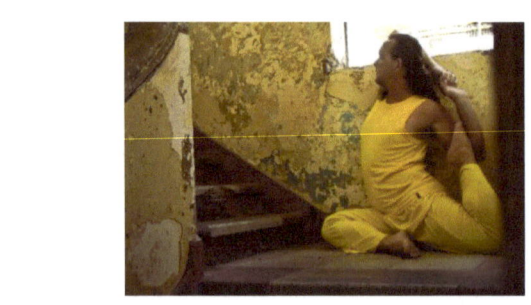

The Backbone of Yoga

Second only to the breath, but also pivotal to the success and safety of your Yoga practice is the spine.

The spine is the secret key to unlock all the potential your body has, to be and function at its optimal best.

The spine protects within it the spinal cord, which is the nerve center of the entire nervous system. Every nerve that communicates the necessary messages to and from the brain to perform every function the organs have in the body, originates in the spinal cord.

The nervous system together with the endocrine system of glands within the body, communicate electrical and chemical signals to wherever they are needed.

When the nerves are disrupted in any way, these signals are weakened or fail to reach their target, and the result can be pain or in the long term, even disease.

A long, strong and flexible spine ensures the integrity of the nervous system, facilitating normal functions within the body, including the prevention and cure of illness.

Stress, which can be physical, chemical or mental, results in tension in the muscles that support the spine. Uneven tension causes misalignments between the vertebrae, and this in turn puts pressure on the nerves, inhibiting their function.

A healthy spine is open and moves freely in five ways. These are forwards, backwards, sideways, twisting and common within each of these others as well, is lengthening.

Keeping awareness of the spine ensures the integrity and effectiveness of any Yoga posture. The aim in any pose is never to compress the spine in any way but to create space between the vertebrae.

Understanding how the spine moves adds a level of depth to your practice that enables you to monitor and adjust your body accordingly.

The idea is to make every pose as big as possible, to take up as much space on the mat or in the room as you can.

Our instincts are to withdraw, use force and work against the body, especially when it doesn't yet do what we think it should.

Always treat your body as gently as possible and using the breath, fill your mind with the courage to let go of whatever stress holds any of your muscles captive.

When bending in any direction, try to observe length in the spine on both the inside of the stretch as well as the outside.

The longer you can envision, and physically extend the spine, the further you will be able to move; the deeper you will be able to go into any posture over time.

Yoga is not about the destination at all though. Having an idea of the direction you are taking, it is important to be with, and accept wherever you are at in the present moment entirely.

Gather Your Bandhas

In order to protect the spine, as well as to direct the proper flow of substances and energy through the body, we employ the use of three specific muscular contractions or "locks".

The first of the three is called Mula Bandha meaning Root Lock, and is a contraction of the pelvic floor muscles.

Imagine the muscles you would use to stop urinating mid-stream. The actual contraction during Yoga is much gentler than that but employs exactly those muscles. It is often sufficient to imagine the contraction just as an intention, moving energy up from the base of the torso into the body.

The Bandhas (Locks) are used slightly differently in Pranayama practices but Mula Bandha is usually exercised on inhalation.

The second of the locks is called Uddiyana Bandha which means Flying Up Lock and is a contraction of the abdominal muscles.

Draw the belly button in towards the spine as much as you can. You should feel a lift of the organs up into the chest. Uddiyana Bandha is again slightly gentler than this but the idea is to create a tender shortening of the space between the lower ribs and the hips.

Contraction of the abdominal muscles has the result of engaging the pelvic floor naturally but, it is the recruitment of the strength in these particular muscles that offer support and protection to the lower back that is of paramount importance.

Uddiyana is engaged on exhalation and allows the body the space and control it needs to move into the postures.

The third lock is called Jalandhara Bandha meaning Net Lock. In Pranayama the chin is tucked into the notch of the collar bones.

In Asana practice the chin is drawn inwards almost to create a double-chin effect.

This lock helps in keeping attention on the Ujjayi breath, as well as lengthening the back of the neck to protect the vertebrae and muscles there.

As upright primates our bodies constantly work against the force of gravity. The careful and deliberate contraction of these three sets of muscles counteracts the effects of gravity on the body.

It becomes easier for blood to reach the heart and for the entire circulatory system to ferry nutrients and waste to and from every cell and tissue.

Energetically, these contractions draw vitality into the body, and stimulate the metabolism, giving us the strength and endurance we need throughout the day.

Take your time to engage them during practice.

Yin & Yang

Yin and Yang refer to the feminine and masculine principles respectively, and more specifically the balance between these.

Yoga is essentially about restoring balance to both body and mind and relies on the use of these energies or principles within Asana practice.

Muscles that are engaged embody the masculine Yang while relaxed muscles embody the feminine Yin.

Experiment with these two within your Yoga practice by using isometric contraction (hardening all of the muscles and the body into statue-like poses) or softening the body, like the bough of a tree in the wind, as you move through your sequence. (Remember to gather your Bandhas always.)

Yang energy will encourage weight-loss and strength-building while Yin energy will aid in detoxifying and toning the body and all its systems.

Sun Salutations

Sun Salutations, known as Surya Namaskara, are where Yoga originally began. The practice involved making obeisance to the ancient sun god, Surya.

A twelve step sequence of postures, together with the chanting of sacred formulas, was established to request long life, health and wealth from the deity.

Today Sun Salutations are usually part of the warming up sequence, so even though we no longer worship the Sun in that way, we pay our respects to the ancient tradition by bringing warmth into the body to prepare ourselves for Asana practice.

Sun Salutations are the very foundation of a sequenced Yoga practice and as such can be practiced entirely on their own.

At any time when we are short of time or unable to attend a formal class, they will suffice quite nicely.

Movement is synchronized with the breathe and when practiced regularly, Sun Salutations help us to discover the natural ebbs and flows within the body, enabling us better internal awareness and intuition regarding our physical and mental states or overall well-being.

As with any Yoga practice care should be taken not to over-exert the body and to adjust or modify positions to ensure comfortable execution of the poses, as per our own body's capability.

A complete Sun Salutation practice consists of five rounds each of two similar sequences of poses, the second slightly more challenging than the first.

The sequences known simply as SUN A and SUN B borrowed from the Ashtanga Yoga tradition follow:

(Adjustments have been made, *shown in green*, to suit the beginner with no prior experience.)

EXHALE	Tadasana	Mountain
INHALE	Urdhva Hastasana	Hands Raised
EXHALE	Uttanasana	Forward Fold
INHALE	Ardha Uttanasana	Half Forward Fold
EXHALE	**Makarasana*	*Crocodile*
INHALE	**Bhujangasana*	*Cobra*
EXHALE	*Makarasana*	*Crocodile*
INHALE	**Bidalasana*	*Cow*
EXHALE	**Marjaryasana*	*Cat*

Repeat For Five Deep Breaths

EXHALE	Adho Mukha Svanasana	Down Dog
INHALE	Ardha Uttanasana	Half Forward Fold
EXHALE	Uttanasana	Forward Fold
INHALE	Urdhva Hastasana	Hands Raised
EXHALE	Tadasana	Mountain

*Makarasana – Lie flat on your belly, hands below shoulders (see p.23)

*Bhujangasana – Resting on the hips, raise the chest off the floor (see p.23)

*Bidalasana / Marjaryasana – On all fours, arch the back while inhaling, and round the back exhaling

Sun Salutation A

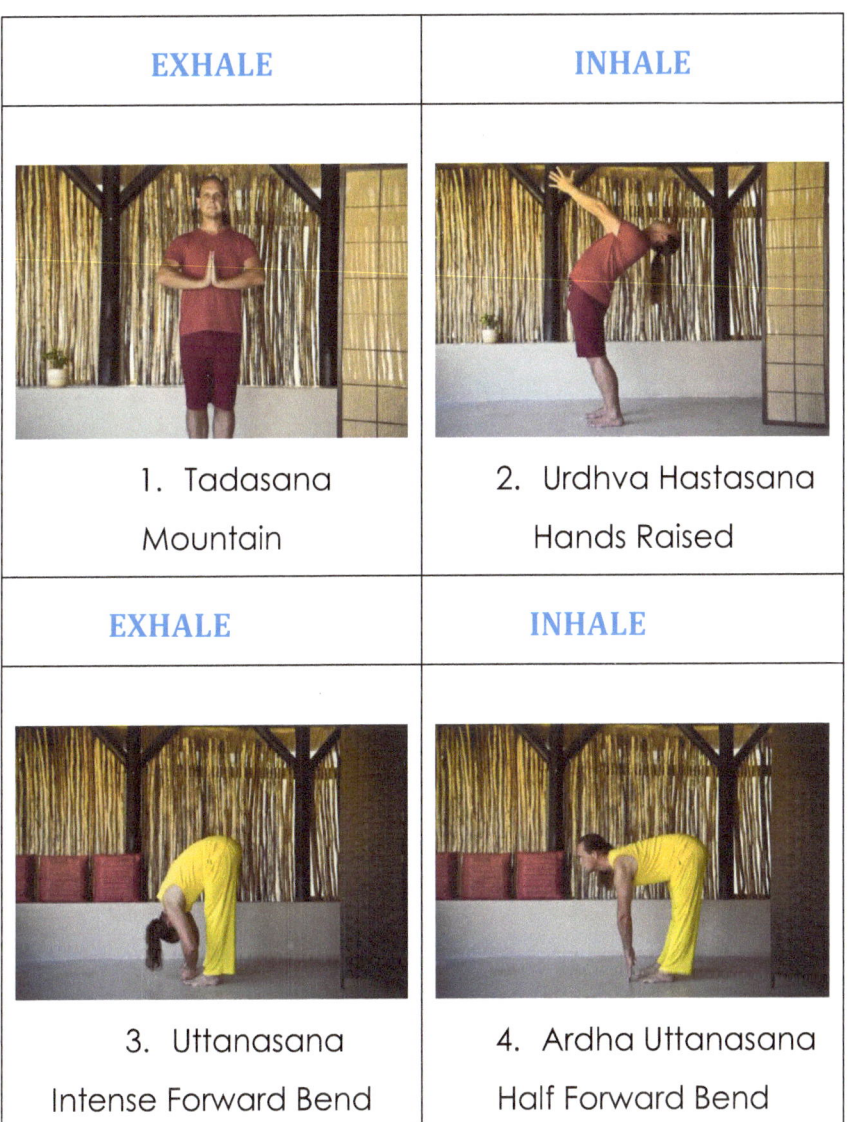

EXHALE	INHALE
1. Tadasana Mountain	2. Urdhva Hastasana Hands Raised

EXHALE	INHALE
3. Uttanasana Intense Forward Bend	4. Ardha Uttanasana Half Forward Bend

Continued...

Continue INHALE	**EXHALE**
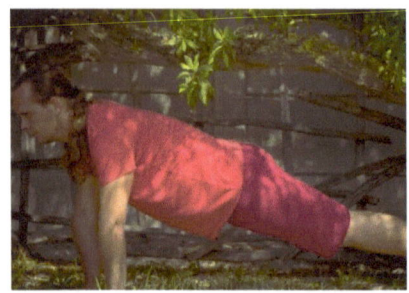	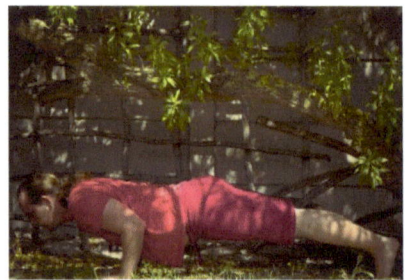
5. Phalakasana High Plank	6. Chataranga Dandasana Four Limbed Staff
INHALE	**EXHALE (Hold x 5 Breaths)**
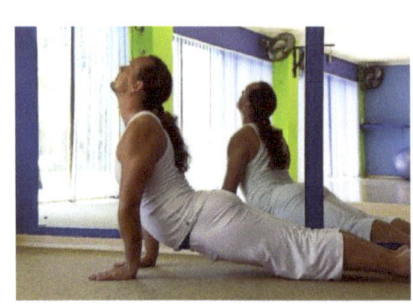	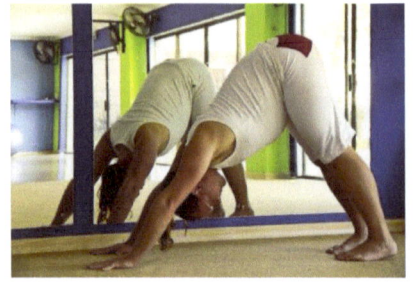
7. Urdhva Mukha Svanasana Upward Facing Dog	8. Adho Mukha Svanasana Downward Facing Dog

Continued...

INHALE	EXHALE
9. Ardha Uttanasana Half Forward Bend	10. Uttanasana Intense Forward Bend
INHALE	**EXHALE**
11. Urdhva Hastasana Hands Raised	12. Tadasana Mountain

Sun Salutation B

EXHALE	Tadasana	Mountain
INHALE	Utkatasana	Fierce
EXHALE	Uttanasana	Forward Fold
INHALE	Ardha Uttanasana	Half Forward Fold
EXHALE	Chataranga Dandasana	Four Limbed Staff
INHALE	Urdhva Mukha Svanasana	Upward Facing Dog
EXHALE	Adho Mukha Svanasana	Down Facing Dog
INHALE	Virabhadrasana I	Warrior 1 (Right)
EXHALE	Chataranga Dandasana	Four Limbed Staff
INHALE	Urdhva Mukha Svanasana	Upward Facing Dog
EXHALE	Adho Mukha Svanasana	Down Facing Dog
INHALE	Virabhadrasana I	Warrior 1 (Left)
EXHALE	Chataranga Dandasana	Four Limbed Staff
INHALE	Urdhva Mukha Svanasana	Upward Facing Dog
EXHALE	Adho Mukha Svanasana	Down Facing Dog

Hold For Five Deep Breaths

(Replace down dog here with five rounds of Cat and Cow stretch if you wish)

INHALE	Ardha Uttanasana	Half Forward Fold
EXHALE	Uttanasana	Forward Fold
INHALE	Utkatasana	Fierce
EXHALE	Tadasana	Mountain

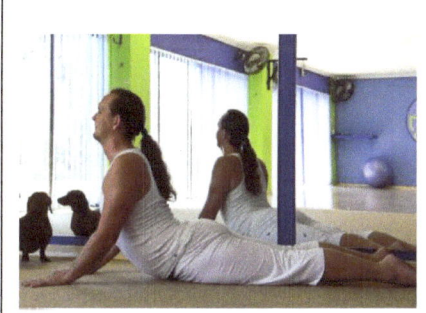

Bhujangasana

Cobra

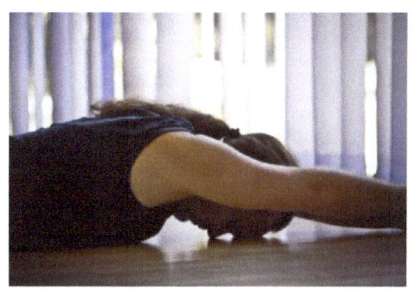

Makarasana

Crocodile

EXHALE	INHALE
1. Tadasana	2. Utkatasana
Mountain	Fierce

EXHALE	INHALE
3. Uttanasana	4. Ardha Uttanasana
Intense Forward Bend	Half Forward Bend

Continued...

Continue INHALE	EXHALE
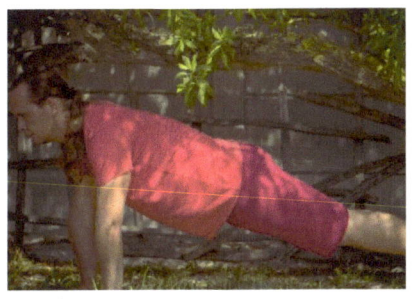	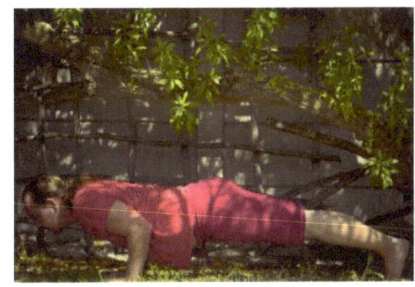
5. Phalakasana High Plank	6. Chataranga Dandasana Four Limbed Staff
INHALE	**EXHALE**
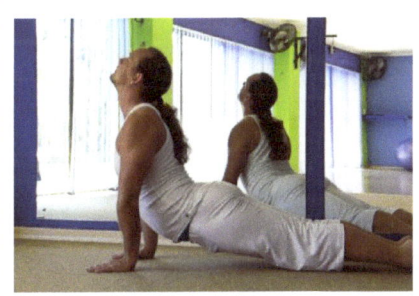	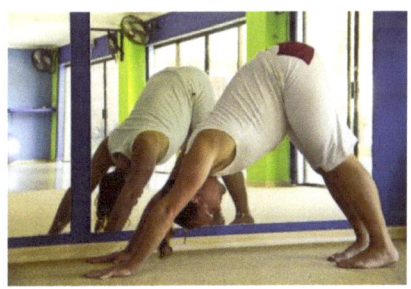
7. Urdhva Mukha Svanasana Upward Facing Dog	8. Adho Mukha Svanasana Downward Facing Dog

Continued...

INHALE	Begin EXHALE
9. Virabhadrasana I Warrior 1 (Right)	10. Phalakasana High Plank
Complete EXHALE	**INHALE**
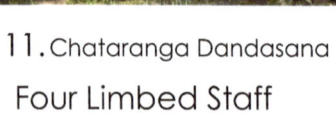	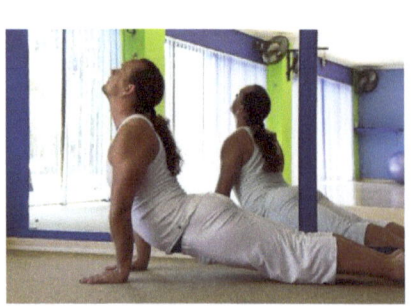
11. Chataranga Dandasana Four Limbed Staff	12. Urdhva Mukha Svanasana Upward Facing Dog

Continued...

EXHALE	INHALE
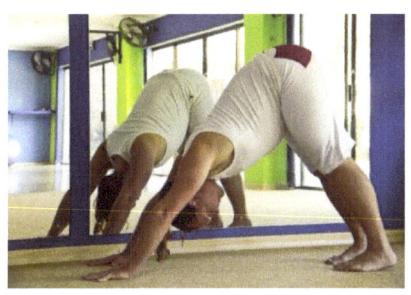	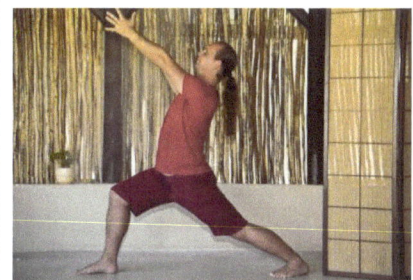
13. Adho Mukha Svanasana Downward Facing Dog	14. Virabhadrasana I Warrior 1 (Left)
Begin EXHALE	**Complete EXHALE**
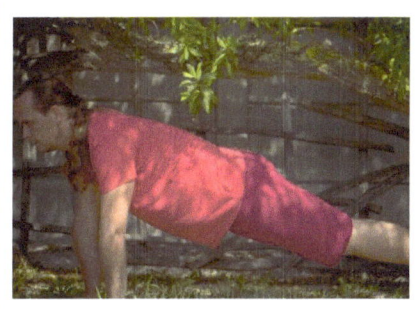	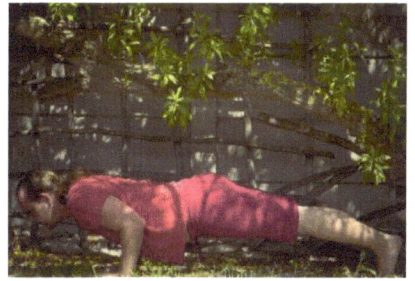
15. Phalakasana High Plank	16. Chataranga Dandasana Four Limbed Staff

Continued...

INHALE	**EXHALE (Hold x 5 Breaths)**
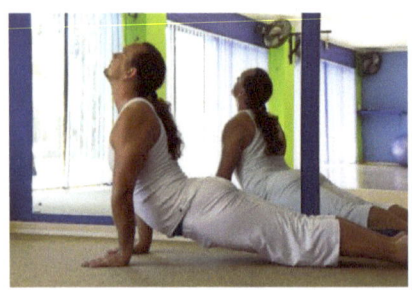	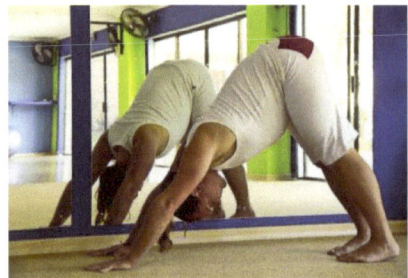
17. Urdhva Mukha Svanasana Upward Facing Dog	18. Adho Mukha Svanasana Downward Facing Dog
INHALE	**EXHALE**
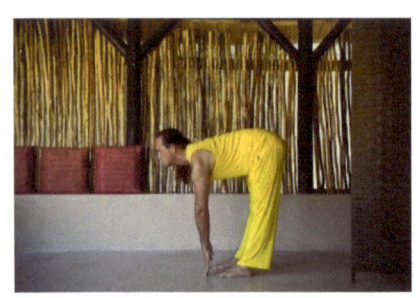	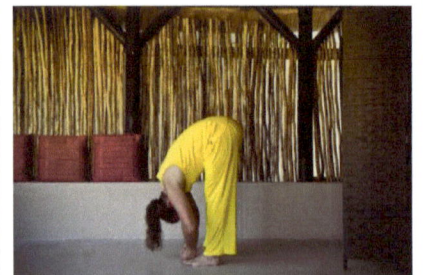
19. Ardha Uttanasana Half Forward Bend	20. Uttanasana Intense Forward Bend

Continued...

INHALE	EXHALE
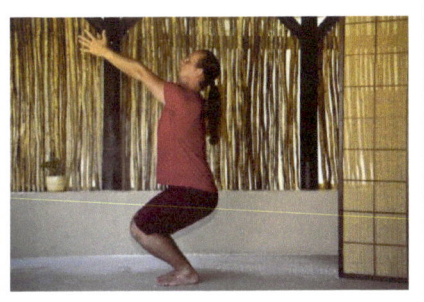	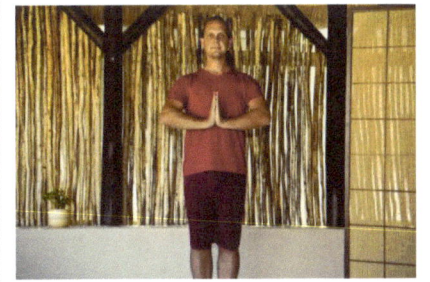
21. Utkatasana Fierce	22. Tadasana Mountain

AUM

Usually chanted at the beginning or end of a yoga class reverences "the Word" that was in the beginning; the sound of all vibrating atoms

"Ah-Oo-Mm" of equal intensity and duration

A Note about Balancing Asanas

These poses can be daunting and challenging, as well as invigorating and satisfying, but they can also be left aside until the body has grown accustomed to a regular Asana practice.

The breath is what really brings the correct kind of focus needed to stabilize the body in balancing poses but it takes some time to master, not relying on brute strength alone.

There are no specific benefits to practicing balances that cannot also be obtained through other Asana but they exist to deepen the experience of centeredness and balance as the body grows stronger, and more adept at its own feedback gained through the realignment taking place during a regular Yoga practice.

The best way to learn is to practice but don't take it too seriously and have fun with these poses.

A Note about Inverted Asanas

Inverted Asanas are mostly described as being the royalty among poses. It is the most nourishing and rejuvenating thing to do for yourself, to turn yourself upside down.

With the head below the heart, the entire body is flushed out, the heart rests not needing to work against gravity, the brain is flooded with nutrients and oxygen while the lymphatic system is drained, detoxifying every tissue.

These poses are also extremely difficult for anyone unprepared (physically and mentally) and also hazardous if practiced incorrectly.

Simple inversions include Rabbit, Down Dog and Shoulder Bridge so there is absolutely no hurry to rush into Head Stands, Shoulder Stands or Arm Balances.

Never attempt these without the guidance of a teacher, who will assess competence and readiness.

Meditation

Meditation was really the reason people began to practice Asana sequences in the first place although we come to the mat for many different reasons today. Originally, Asana was employed to prepare the body, keeping it lithe and strong enough, to be able to sit for extended periods in meditation.

Meditation can be deep, complex and religious yet it can also be simple and secular, and still have profound benefits to our overall well-being.

Classes may sometimes end with Pranayama exercises but for the sake of the beginner, the simplest method to still the mind is turning awareness towards the breath.

With practice we continuously develop greater internal awareness of both the mind and body. Taking any comfortable seat, with spine erect and chest open, we direct our attention inwards.

There are an untold number of ways to meditate.

One is to feel the rise and fall of the chest as you breathe in and breathe out, noting the quality and depth of each breath without influence upon it of any kind.

Another method is to count the length of the inhalation in seconds and then to either count the same amount on exhalation or to extend the exhalation somewhat. A longer exhale causes a relaxation response in the body and can aid with anxiety or insomnia.

The breath can be counted up to ten, with inhalation and exhalation equaling one. Then it can be counted back from ten to one again. This is slightly more difficult to do but as such develops our powers of concentration and can aid with focused work or study.

All the while the mind will be full of thoughts. The trick is to pay them no attention. Simply allow thoughts to enter and leave the mind.

Take a step back and become an observer to your thinking mind, without participating in the thought process, as far as possible.

Relaxation

Relaxation, after the breath and the spine, is the next most crucial part of your Yoga practice.

Relaxation should constitute at least one third of your entire practice and should not be less than an absolute minimum of three to eight minutes at the end of a class. The longer the better! Some of the relaxation occurs when returning to foundational poses such as Mountain or Staff during Asana practice.

The magic happens in Savasana (Corpse Pose) as the mind and body are settled, surrendering the weight of both to the mat and ground beneath it.

All the systems of the body are aligned and in communication with one another, bringing the whole body into its natural homeostatic state.

Balance is brought to the chemical messengers of the endocrine system.

Healing and repair, after exertion, begin to take place.

It is often the hardest part of a Yoga class, to remain still instead of moving. A hundred and one pressing matters to be dealt with after class begin to assert their presence in your thoughts.

You've put in the hard work until this point though, and it is well worth it to allow the benefits of proper, induced relaxation to have their effects on your mind and body.

Relaxation is the antithesis of everything else we do to ourselves throughout our day and an essential component of Yoga to ensure balance for rejuvenation and restoration.

Always try to be the last person to leave the class or the last to sit up before final greetings.

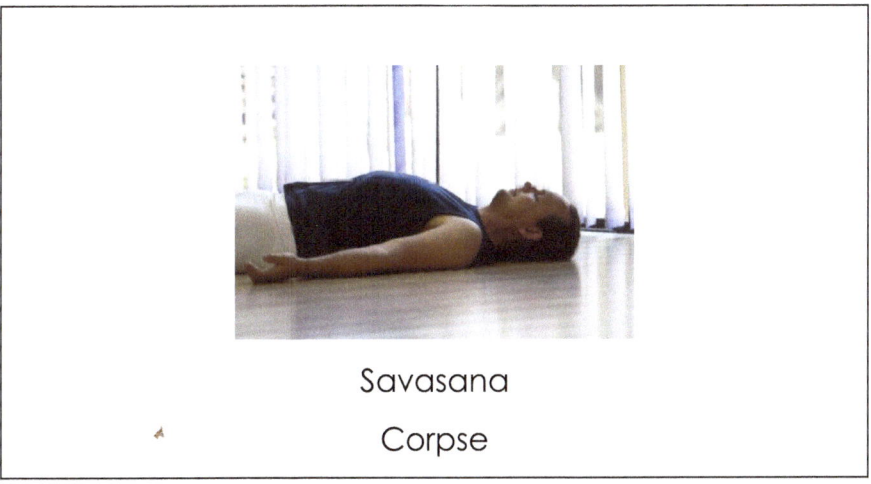

Savasana

Corpse

Role of the Yoga Teacher

Another word you may likely hear in a Yoga class is Drishti, meaning focal point. These are used to add another layer to your Asana practice by directing your attention to areas of the room or specific parts of the body.

As a beginner, your Drishti will probably be the teacher at the front of the class so there is no need to pay too much attention to it at the start of your Yoga practice.

The teacher is however, a voice in the background to your practice, a guide more than an authority.

It is important to cultivate a sense of self-responsibility for your practice and to develop awareness in response to your own body of what feels right to you.

Many teachers, trained in different schools may have varying techniques and explanations. None are explicitly right or wrong and the onus is on you to choose one preference or another.

Yoga teaching is an informal qualification granted on some academic merit, years of practice and self-study. A lot of the knowledge that your teacher shares with you will likely be based on personal experience and intuition.

Bearing that in mind, it is of utmost importance that you always inform your teacher of any medical condition (including pregnancy) or injury that you may have. It is also wise to consult a medical professional before beginning a Yoga practice should there be any doubt.

Your Yoga teacher has experienced the many wonderful and amazing benefits that Yoga has to offer and for this reason has endeavored to share that with you. You should feel free to be open and honest with your teacher at all times in order that he or she is better equipped to tailor instructions to suit your own needs.

Try many different teachers and choose one that fits your own temperament. Your Yoga teacher is bound to be a long term companion on your journey towards holistic wellness.

Simple Yoga Practice

5 Minutes Balasana – Child's Pose or

Savasana – Corpse Pose

10 Minutes Surya Namaskara A – Sun Salutation A x 5

15 Minutes Surya Namaskara B – Sun Salutation B x 5

5 Minutes Bhavana – Meditation

Sit in any comfortable seated position

10 Minutes Savasana – Corpse Pose

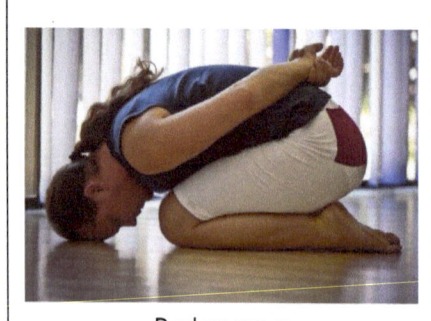

Balasana
Childs Pose

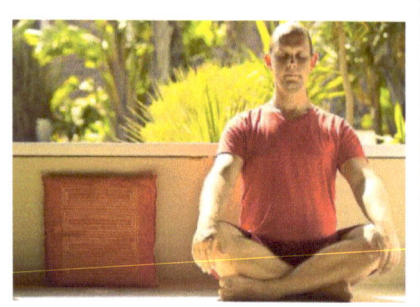

Sukhasana
Easy Seated

Glossary

Asana – Pose / Posture / Seat lit.

Ashtanga Yoga – Sequence Based Tradition

Bandha – Lock / Bind

Drishti – Gaze / Point of Awareness / Focal Point

Hatha Yoga – Therapeutic Tradition

Iyengar Yoga – Alignment Based Tradition

Jalandhara Bandha – Net Lock / Chin Tucking

Mula Bandha – Root Lock / Pelvic Floor Lift

Namaste – (The Divine is Omnipresent)

Pranayama – Breathing / Energy Expanding lit.

Surya Namaskara – Sun Salutations

Uddiyana Bandha – Flying Up Lock / Abdominal Lift

Ujjayi Pranayama – Victorious Breath Technique

Vinyasa Yoga – Flowing Tradition

Yoga – Training / Union / Yoking lit.

Notes

....

....

....

....

....

....

....

....

....

....

....

....

....

Namaste

"The Divine in me greets the Divine in you"

www.ingramcontent.com/pod-product-compliance
Lightning Source LLC
Chambersburg PA
CBHW040316010626
45792CB00022B/582